Hormone Diet: How To Balance Your Hormones And Boost Your Metabolism

Hormone Diet Reloaded: The Lifestyle Changing Guide

By: Anna Gracey

ISBN-13: 978-1480173491

TABLE OF CONTENTS

Anna Gracey

Publishers Notes

Disclaimer

This publication is intended to provide helpful and informative material. It is not intended to diagnose, treat, cure, or prevent any health problem or condition, nor is intended to replace the advice of a physician. No action should be taken solely on the contents of this book. Always consult your physician or qualified health-care professional on any matters regarding your health and before adopting any suggestions in this book or drawing inferences from it.

The author and publisher specifically disclaim all responsibility for any liability, loss or risk, personal or otherwise, which is incurred as a consequence, directly or indirectly, from the use or application of any contents of this book.

Any and all product names referenced within this book are the trademarks of their respective owners. None of these owners have sponsored, authorized, endorsed, or approved this book.

Always read all information provided by the manufacturers' product labels before using their products. The author and publisher are not responsible for claims made by manufacturers.

Paperback Edition 2012

Manufactured in the United States of America

DEDICATION

I want to dedicate this book to my mother, she has been an inspiration in my life since day one and I would not be the woman I am today without her guidance. Thanks Mum!

CHAPTER 1- WHAT EXACTLY IS A HORMONE?

The chemicals that transport messages from the glands to the cells in organ or tissues of the body are known as hormones. These hormones also regulate the levels of chemicals in the bloodstream to assist with the balance or stability in the body (homeostasis).

There are two kinds of chemicals, peptides and steroids. Hormone is a derivative of the Greek word which means "to spur on." This basically explains how the hormones function as catalysts for changes in chemicals at the cellular level which are required for energy, development and growth.

How Does It Work

As a part of the endocrine system, the hormones are manufactured by glands. The chemicals flow freely in the bloodstream, waiting for a target cell to locate it.

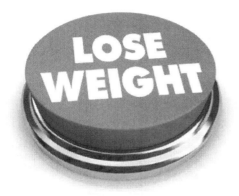

This cell contains a receptor which can be triggered by a particular type of hormone, and the cell will then begin to carry out a specific function. For example certain genes might get stimulated. The paracrine hormone acts on cells that are close by but unrelated while the autocrine hormone works on the cells of the secreting gland.

Steroids

Generally speaking, steroids are sex hormones which are directly linked to fertility and sexual maturation. These steroids are made from cholesterol either from the ovaries or ovaries (gonads) or the adrenal glands in the body after birth or the placenta while the baby is still in the mother's womb.

An example of a steroid hormone is cortisol. It helps to break down any tissue that is damaged so that it can be replaced. These steroids will spur the fertility cycles and physical development from pubescence right through to old age. If the body is not processing the right hormones then it can be supplemented with progesterone and estrogen.

Peptides

These are responsible for controlling other functions like the concentration of sugar in the blood and sleep. They are made up of the long strings in amino acids and are often referred to as protein hormones. HGH (human growth hormone) helps the body to burn muscle and fat. Insulin, another peptide hormone triggers the process of converting sugar into cellular energy.

Homeostasis

Homeostasis is managed by negative feedback cycles and the main goal of the body is to maintain the levels of certain chemicals for a particular period of time. when there negative feedback is employed it causes a change in current conditions which then triggers a response to get it all back to normal. So for example when the temperature falls in a room, the thermostat will turn the heat on and then turn it off when the temperature is restored.

CHAPTER 2- FOOD AND HORMONES

You can have a beef cow that grows twenty percent faster than other cows or a salmon that gets to a size that can be sold in the market twice as fast or even a dairy cow that produces fifteen percent more milk. The question is what is common in these animals?

As a result of genetic engineering (salmon) or implants or injections (cows) they have higher levels of synthetic of growth or sex hormones.

Many may wonder if these synthetic hormones pose any danger to the individuals that drink the milk or eat the food. The food industry says it has no effect and the FDA (Food and Drug Administration) agrees to a certain extent (there is an issue with the cows).

The Food and Drug Administration is responsible for regulating the use of hormones on livestock and they have not yet made the judgment on whether or not they will allow the sale of genetically engineered salmon or any other animal. Vegetables and fruits have been genetically engineered for years.

The stamp of approval from the FDA is not really going to serve as a form of reassurance for those that are concerned that these surplus hormones can trigger health problems, early puberty in females and cause certain types of cancer. For quite a number of years, public health experts and consumer advocates have battled to reduce the use of hormones in cows.

The thing is that it is not really clear if these hormones are really bad for us. Not a lot of research has been done on the effects that they can have, partially due to the fact that it is hard to distinguish the effects of the added hormones from the natural as well as the other components in meat and milk. The skeptical will but organic but there really isn't any proof that it is that much safer.

The FDA approved a synthetic cow hormone that increased the production of milk when it was injected into dairy cows in nineteen ninety three. This is known as rBGH (recombinant bovine growth hormone). There are groups that have been questioning the safety of this since it was approved. The genetic engineering of salmon is also questioned.

The recombinant bovine growth hormone by itself has no discernible effect on humans and poses no threat to one's health. The same applies to the hormone used on the salmon.

The main fear that persons have is that this manipulation of hormones will increase the levels of another hormone the IGF (insulin growth factor that can clone the effects on HGH in a negative way. In fact it has been shown through research that the levels of IGF in rBGH treated cows are ten times higher.

These higher levels of IGF have been linked to prostrate, breast and other cancers in persons. in a study done in two thousand and four, patients that had high levels of insulin growth factor had approximately a sixty five percent greater risk of premenopausal breast cancer and a fifty percent higher risk of prostate cancer than other persons with normal levels.

A number of factors including fat intake, smoking and genes all contribute to the presence of these cancers. The thing is that a part of the equation does include the levels of IGF especially in the incidences of prostate cancer.

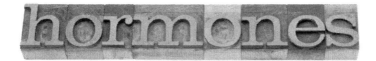

Though the consumption of copious amounts of dairy and milk have been proven to increase the levels if IGF, it is not necessarily related to the level of IGF found in foods. This is due to the fact that the levels of IGF in dairy products is not as much as the amounts found naturally in the body whether the cow is rBGH treated or not.

Just to acquire the amount of IGF that can be found in the digestive tract and the saliva you would have to consume approximately ninety five quarts of milk. This is what a Pennsylvania State University professor of dairy and animal science names Terry Etherton Ph. D. had to say. This professor is also an author of a blog on food biotechnology. You would also have to consume approximately one hundred and seventy three ounce servings of salmon.

The question is if the levels of IGF in milk are insignificant, how then does the consumption of milk cause an increase in the levels of IGF. Generally speaking milk along with the non-IGF hormones, minerals, sugar and proteins that it contains can somehow cause the human body to produce more on its own. This is what was stated by Dr. Willett.

Early Puberty and Sex Hormones

The thing to note is that IGF is not the only hormone that is found in food. Farmers have also been making use of sex hormones to fatten up cattle since as early as the nineteen fifties, estrogen being the most popular choice. Almost all of the beef cows in the United States apart from the organic ones get an implant in their ear that delivers estradiol (a form of estrogen) along with a mix of five other hormones. The interesting point to note is that these hormones are not given to pigs and chickens as they do not have the same effect.

A major concern is that the hormones can trigger puberty at an earlier age in children as they are going into pubescence at an earlier age than they did one or two generations ago. The reasons are still being determined for this.

There is however a researcher at the Pennsylvania State University in the Department of Dairy and Animal Science named Ann Macrina Ph.D. that states that the level of estrogen that meat contains is miniscule to the amount that we have in our bodies.

A three ounce portion of beef for example from a cow that was treated with estrogen has less than a billionth of a gram which is approximately one hundred times lower than the amount in males and four hundred times lower than the amount in females.

In spite if this however, Dr. Willet states that these small amounts of estrogen can affect boys and girls that are prepubescent. It is based on the fact that for a young girl that is not yet producing these hormones on her own it is quite a bit.

A study done in two thousand and nine found that children who got their source of protein from animal sources went into puberty approximately seven months earlier than those that did not have as much.

According to Thomas Renner Ph.D. it does not really matter if it is meat, cheese or milk; all the proteins from animals affect the human

IGF system. He is a professor at the German based research Institute of Child Nutrition and an author of the study.

In spite of this hormones that are added to the supply of food are most likely not the biggest contributors to the early onset of puberty. The likelihood of this comes from milk, meat and similar foods as they are rich in nutrients, calories and protein. This is based on a study done in nineteen ninety seven by adjunct professor at the School of Public Health at the University of North Carolina Marcia Herman-Giddens.

In spite of this she does warn that more research has to be done to find all of the factors that are involved.

She cites an example using the increasing rate of persons that are obese and overweight. She also mentions the lack of exercise, high calorie drinks and processed foods that drive them. She thinks that this is a major contributing factor to the early onset of puberty as the fat cells will trigger the production of estrogen). There are also external factors such as plastics, flame retardants, pesticides and other chemicals that can disrupt the hormones.

Is Organic Necessary?

The USDA (U.S. Department of Agriculture) certified dairy and beef products come with the assurance that the cows received no sex hormones or rBGH. They also tend to cost more. The question is whether or the extra spend is worth it.

According to Dr. Willett it is not. This doctor is in favor of not eating a lot of meat in the first place and recommends no more than two servings on a weekly basis. As the consumption is not much it really does not matter if is it organic or not.

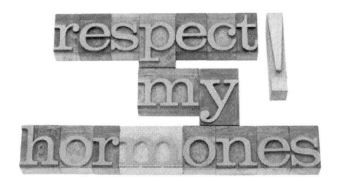

The same type of advice is proffered by Dr. Willett on organic dairy products. On the flip side there are other experts like Herman-Giddens that do not recommend milk that is from rBGH treated cows as it can trigger higher levels of IGF. It also does not have any increased level of benefits than regular milk.

The recommendation is made to cut back on the consumption of dairy instead of option for the more expensive organic option. All of this is said despite the fact that three servings of dairy are recommended per day by the USDA.

Another professor, Bruce Chassy, Ph.D., from the University of Illinois states that the information circulated by persons who do organic farming is far from correct. He in fact supports the use of synthetic hormones as they do have some benefits. Farmers will be able to get the same amount of milk with fewer cows and these cows will also be better for suited for the environment.

He also states that the genetically engineered salmon does not consume as much feed as the regular fish. The fears he said are based on the true value of hormone free and organic. Those are the main selling points for organic farmers.

He is of the belief that a lot of farms do not use rBGH as they feel that consumers do not want the milk. He also feels that the genetically engineered salmon will set off marketing campaigns for fish that is hormone. He finds it absurd as all milk and meat does contain hormones.

Let us now look at how certain foods help the body.

Food that help to cool the body:

Papaya-contains no sodium, great digestive and liver cleanser and has high levels of iron and vitamins A and C

Tea, borage oil or black currant

Watermelon-low in calories and has high levels of vitamin C- perfect for individuals that are watching their weight.

Raspberry- high in vitamin c, iron and fiber

Broccoli-high levels of vitamins A and C as well as folate

Persimmons and cherries- high levels of vitamin C

Brown rice-high levels of magnesium and niacin and also source of zinc, fiber and protein.

Yam/Sweet potato-great source of potassium and vitamin C; also great source of carbohydrates for energy

Foods that help when you feel cold:

Grains, meats, ginger and cardamom

Anna Gracey

Black tea with milk (iron)

Cardamom, ginger, meats and grains

Management of Weight:

To lose weight- kiwifruit, grapefruit and boysenberries are low in calories, contain fiber and have high levels of vitamin C

To gain weight- consume nuts and grains that have high mineral and vitamin content.

Sex-Drive:

Circulation can be improved with Omega 3, 6 and 9 oils

Rosemary also helps with circulation

Cardamom works well as an aphrodisiac.

Mood Stabilizer:

Green tea

Foods packed with B complex vitamins

Lemon balm, chamomile and lavender

Jerusalem artichoke-great source of thiamine, iron and potassium

Mango-high levels of vitamins A and C- great for treating depression

Memory:

Keep levels of sugar balanced

Consume walnuts, oily fish and flaxseed oil for omega 3 fatty acids

Hormone Diet

Consume organic vegetables, seeds, free-range eggs to get omega 6 fatty acids

Ginkgo biloba herb and rosemary tea

Exhaustion:

Consume dark leafy greens, mushrooms, lima beans, seaweed and brown rice

Asparagus- contains vitamins E and C

Tea with rosemary, ginger, lemon and ginseng

Consume dandelion, beetroot and cherries (iron rich foods).

CHAPTER 3- A HEALTHY HORMONE DIET

I personally have learned how to keep my hormones balanced over the past year through taking nutritional supplements and make changes to the diet. The problems I had with chronic fatigue are gone and the melasma is eighty to ninety percent cleared.

Top Five Tips to Naturally Balance Hormones

Consume a Lot of Good Fats

Diets that are low in fat are the primary reason why women of all ages are experiencing issues with their hormones. These hormones are made from cholesterol. In short if there is not enough cholesterol in the diet, the body will not be able to produce any hormones.

What exactly are the good fats? The typical fats have been in existence for a while. These include olive oil, palm oil, coconut oil, beef tallow, lard, coconut milk, whole milk, egg yolks, cream and butter.

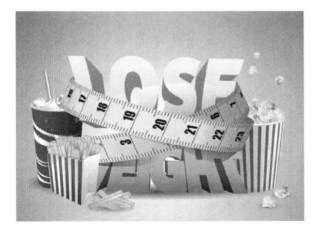

Fats that are bad ought to be avoided; these include hydrogenated oils, cottonseed oil, soybean oil, vegetable oil and canola oil.

Stay Away From Soy

I am of the opinion that a major reason why there are so many hormonal issues nowadays is a result of the rise of the level of soy that we eat. Soy is classified as a goitrogen which inhibits the uptake of iodine in the body. In females this iodine is stored in the ovaries, breasts and the thyroid gland.

A deficiency in iodine leads to disorders in the thyroid. This includes thyroid cancer, hyperthyroidism, hypothyroidism and goiters, ovarian cancer, breast cancer and cysts in the ovaries and breasts.

You may feel as if you are not consuming a lot of soy as you don't eat tofu or drink soy milk. The thing is that nowadays soy can be found in almost anything.

A lot of restaurants utilize soybean to cook and a lot of the processed and packaged foods contain soy lecithin and soybean oil. A lot of the dairy and meat that we consume comes from animals that are fed with soy. A lot of salad dressings and mayonnaise also include soybean oil.

It is fine to consume soy in moderate amounts or use it as a condiment providing it is fermented naturally (naturally fermented natto, tempeh, miso and soy sauce). It is better to avoid packaged and processed foods that have soy in it.

Don't Forget the Minerals

A lot of us do not have enough minerals in our bodies. The phytic acid that can be found in whole grains like whole wheat and oats rob the body of minerals except they are sprouted or soaked properly.

Minerals are extremely important when it comes to balancing hormones. As an example if your body does not have enough zinc, you will not produce the right amount of testosterone. It is essential for maintaining a healthy sex drive.

As a trace mineral, iodine is one thing that most us of lack. A thing to note is that the Japanese have the lowest rate of breast cancer. I think that this is as a result of the fact that copious quantities of iodine are consumed by them as seaweed or fish broth. A point to note is that they do not eat as much soy based products they do fish and seaweed.

The Japanese tend to consume miso soup with each meal. Traditional miso soup is made using bonito broth and this broth is fish based. As the fish used in small, the entire fish is put in the broth, heads included.

The head of the fish contains the thyroid gland and this is where the iodine is. A point to note is that if you are preparing fish broth, the head of the fish should be included so you can benefit from the iodine. The miso soup also has seaweed in it which has high levels of iodine as well.

If you are not having this soup on a daily basis it is recommended that you take a supplement to get the right doses of iodine. Lugol or Iodoral, two supplements can provide the iodine needed.

I recommend that you find out how much iodine you have in your body before taking any supplements. A test can be ordered online. If you have hyperthyroidism or Hashimoto's you should not be taking iodine supplements.

A also take zinc and magnesium as well. I know that those levels are low in my body. I also take a supplement with multi minerals.

Why Maca?

I began to take this in the fall of last year for about a six week period. I took about half a teaspoon daily. The outcomes that I got are great.

The symptoms that I had with PMS and cramps are no longer there and the melasma also reduced drastically since I started my maca regimen.

I even had a time when I was not on maca for a couple of months as my supply was finished and I did not get back on my routine quickly. Surprisingly I lost none of the benefits for a while but I did have to go back on it when I got the cramps.

Maca is classified as an herb that is adaptogenic. This merely means that it helps to maintain hormonal balance. If your levels of progesterone are low, it will help the body to produce more and if your levels of cortisol are high, it can be lowered with maca.

Stay Away From Caffeine, Sugar and White Flour

Caffeine, white sugar and flour are not good for the adrenal glands.

A better option is to eat bread that is sprouted instead of bread made from white flour. This flour can be bromated which inhibits uptake of iodine.

Stick to the natural sweeteners as well like stevia, palm sugar, maple syrup, sucanat, rapadura, molasses and honey. .

CHAPTER 4- THE MASTER FAT CONTROL HORMONE

"Leptos", a Greek word which means thin, is where the word leptin originated. This hormone dubbed "the hunger hormone" according to New York's Columbia University professor of medicine Dr. Steven Heymsfield has a great effect on the expenditure of energy and the intake of food.

Produced in the fat cells, leptin sends signals to the brain to indicate whether or not the body has enough fat or stores of energy. The hormone will send signals of satiety to the hypothalamus to let us know when we should stop eating. This is what Dr. Julio Licinio, a University of California Los Angeles School of Medicine professor of psychiatry and medicine states.

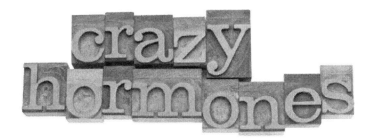

Everyone has leptin with the exception of three cousins in Turkey Zeynep Fakili, Bayrum Donsek and Elif Fakili that are leptin deficient as the result of a genetic mutation. When there is no leptin the body will never get the message that the body is sufficiently satiated. As a result the brain will think that the body is in need of food. As a result of this the Turkish cousins constantly eat and rang from two hundred plus pongs to over three hundred pounds and they never feel full.

Dr. Licinio flew these cousins to his university to take part in some clinical trials that were funded by the National Institutes of Health. They were injected with leptin daily for over a ten month period and the results of this were noted.

The results were incredible as they stopped eating voraciously and began to lose weight. They were not put on any special diet but ended up eating less as a result of the effects of leptin on their appetite.

Apart from that leptin also stimulates what we do physically so the levels of activity increased for these Turkish cousins and over time the excess weight began to disappear. In a one year period they lost approximately half of it.

The Ideal Subjects

In nineteen ninety five when researchers at the Rockefeller University injected leptin into fat mice, they saw that the mice lost weight quickly. When leptin was discovered it opened up the door to weight loss paradise. The only problem was that it did not work the same way for humans as it did for animals.

This is due to the fact that the levels of leptin vary from one person to the next. Dr. Licinio was aware of this and stated that when excess hormones are given, it may not have a distinct effect so it is a bit more difficult to tell what the hormone really does.

The way to get to the bottom of the mystery and the role it plays in controlling weight is to start at the beginning and look for individuals that had no leptin at all. This is where the Turkish cousin came in. Finding them was akin to finding a rare gem.

With their help Licinio was able note the real effects that the hormone had when administered. When leptin is not present in the body at all, it leads to a rare form of obesity. The main aim was to get a better understanding of the effects leptin had on body weight.

Foods That Inhibits Leptin

The body is not able to consume leptin, it has to produce it. In spite of this, foods rich in omega 3 fatty acids like sardines, tuna, salmon, snapper, halibut, cod, fish oil, flax seed oil and flax seed can lower the levels of leptin and increase metabolism in the body.

Research

Scientists at the Mayo Clinic looked at the levels of leptin in two African tribes. One tribe ate mostly vegetables while the other ate fish. It was found that the tribe that ate vegetables had five times more leptin than those that ate fish. This indicates that the consumption of fish can lower the levels of leptin.

Example of Meals

If you are not sure of how to incorporate fish in your meals you can try using cod, halibut or tuna to make fish tacos along with tomatoes, lettuce, guacamole and salsa. You can also season the fish with a bit of lemon pepper, bake it and serve it with asparagus on the side over rice.

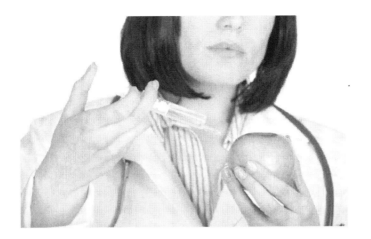

CHAPTER 5- THE FAT-STORING HORMONE

Noted below are the top five hormones that you should be aware of if you want to learn the ways that you can balance your hormones.

Insulin

When there is insulin in the blood stream as a result of sugars and carbs, your body can store fat. This is the main reason why, when you are trying to lose body fat and get healthy, it is recommended that the cabs and proteins are consumed separately. This is to not only rest the stomach but also to balance the hormones (lower body fat).

Keeping added sugars and grain based carbs separated from protein and fat and not consuming them more that once per day within a two hour period can really help to regulate the levels of insulin available to store fat. When the levels of insulin are balanced with regard to other hormones, the process of balancing the fat to muscle ratio in the balance can begin.

The point is that it is not that we cannot consume carbs and proteins together. If you are in perfect health it can be done without any difficulty. As it relates to the glycemic index meals that are properly combined will help to maintain the levels of blood sugar.

There is a challenge however. The modern way of consuming food and the constant eating has led to un-digestion and indigestion. This results in severe deficiencies in Omega 3, minerals and nutrients. This way of eating also leads to addictions to drugs, alcohol, carbs and stimulants which is originally caused by rotting and fermenting food in the stomach which leads to bacterial and yeast problems, diabetes, weight gain and belly fat.

Limiting and separating the consumption of carbohydrates is a great method of allowing the stomach to heal by working with the way the body is built, lowering cholesterol (low density lipids), cutting down on excess body fat and regulating the production of insulin.

As soon as the hormones in the stomach are healthy, the system will be better able to process carbs and meat together without a problem.

Cortisol and Adrenaline

These hormones help to store fat but also help to relieve stress. The levels of these hormones tend to increase when a stressful situation arises, which leads to an increase in the demand for resources or serves as a backup plan for the production of insulin. Bothe these hormones have to be regulated to ensure that the heart is protected and to prevent additional fat from being stored in the abdominal area.

Estrogen

This is another hormone that we tend to have high amounts of. This estrogen is made when we produce hormones naturally, but we also consume phyto-estrogens through the consumption of soy products. Soy for example can have a drastic effect on disease as a result of the fake hormone reaction in both the female and male body. Apart from that there tend to be a lot of hormones in commercial meat.

Clearly, getting rid of the consumption of estrogen is the primary step that you can take to restore balance. You can also stop consuming soy products and opt for better dairy and meat choices. Regulation of this cycle will have a noticeable effect on your overall health.

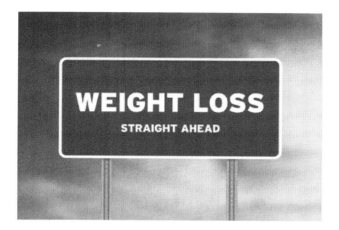

Another issue that we can link to the discussion of estrogen is the other counterpart necessary for balance-progesterone. When cortisol and adrenaline, two fat storing hormones get elevated and are eventually used up, progesterone serves as a backup. This hormone can be used by the body to facilitate the production of the other hormones.

This is a temporary fix however, as when we exist on the adrenaline rush that we get from stimulants and stress, progesterone is always used to assist the adrenal production. When this happens, the levels of the temperature regulating, fat storing estrogen will fluctuate leading to the onset of all types of dysfunction and disease.

Thyroid

This is the most well known fat storing hormone. The thyroid tends to be the first gland that is checked when there is a complaint of weight gain. Suffice it to say that it should be the last on the list of things that need to be regulated to get the desired results.

In practically every case, if the emphasis is placed on balancing the hormonal cycle, you will soon realize that the thyroid hormones do not need to be regulated.

The exception to the rule is surgery. Other than that, you can have an optimistic outlook on how the thyroid works as well as the optimal functioning metabolic process.

CHAPTER 6- THE FAT-REMOVING HORMONE

As you take a walk on a nice sunny day what is it that is on your mind? The breeze, the sun and how it feels to free up those limbs. The last thing that you should be thinking of is what is happening in your body.

Anytime you exercise, the body chemistry gets altered in ways that we are just beginning to understand. Over the last twenty years, scientists have found natural molecules that have an effect on our metabolism and appetite and our weight. They are not only discovering that these molecules have an effect on weight but also trigger other health benefits.

According to Harvard Medical School professor Dr. Anthony Komaroff, the cell muscles require a source of energy when they are exercised. These muscles get energy by burning sugar and fat that they get from the blood. This is something that has been know for quite a while but that is not the entire story.

Irisin

A research team led by Harvard Medical School Professor Dr. Bruce Spiegelman, published a new study in "Journal Nature" in January of two thousand and twelve. The study was conducted on mice but can be applied to humans. It showed that a hormone known as Irisin was produced when the muscles are exercised.

Dr. Komaroff explains that Irisin is transported through the body via the blood and has an effect on fat cells. He indicates that fat cells store body fat and that most of the cells that store fat are white fat cells.

Brown Fat vs. White Fat

The question is why do we store fat? When we consume more calories than we burn, the excess calories don't just disappear. They get stored as fat. Bear in mind that our ancestors did not eat like us. They ate when they could get food so they had to have a source of energy. Most of it came from fat that was stored after they ate.

Studies done at the other institutions including the Harvard Medical School in two thousand and nine shows that we have both brown and white fat cells, according to Dr. Komaroff if the aim is to lose excess weight then the level of white cells have to be decreased while the level of brown fat cells are increased.

This is the effect that Irisin had on mice. The Irisin made from new brown fat cells continue to burn calories when exercise is complete. It does get better.

The Other Benefits of Irisin

We have been aware for a while that doing moderate exercise on a regular basis will prevent us from type 2 diabetes. A program that included some form of exercise can lower the risk of the development of type 2 diabetes by up to sixty percent. This is more effective than medicines currently on the market. How exactly is this possible? Irisin may be holding the answer. Apart from the effect that it has on the creation of brown fat cells, it also helps to overcome or prevent resistance to insulin which can cause type 2 diabetes.

Even though the studies that Dr. Spiegelman conducted were on mice, he discovered that humans do have Irisin as well. Though it is yet to be proven, the effects on humans are probably similar.

The studies are extremely interesting and help to foster an understanding of how the body works. This discovery can have beneficial and practical applications. In theory Irisin could be the solution to allow us to keep the threat of diabetes low and help us maintain healthy body weight.

The fact is however, that products with similar attributes are no longer being considered. Irisin is not a manufactured pharmaceutical but a part of the natural chemical makeup of the body. This can make it much more effective and less likely to have any side effects so there is reason to be excited about it.

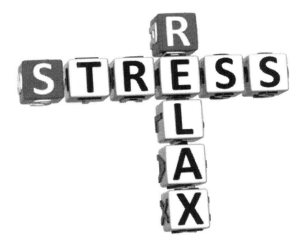

One has to however think of the environment and how it has an effect on behavior. This is the factor that will determine how much we eat and *how much we exercise* and in the long run how much we weigh. According to Dr. Komaroff the solution lies in exercise.

CHAPTER 7- – IRISIN FOOD AND EXERCISE DIET – KEY TO CONTROLLING AND BURNING FAT

If it has the effects that hormones think it will, it will be a vital discovery for the health. Reducing the levels of white fat can have a great effect on the homeostasis of glucose, lowering the risk of type 2 diabetes as well as several other health concerns linked with metabolic syndrome.

Research is required to sort out how the human fat tissue will respond. The question of whether we need to lose white fat tissue and develop more brown tissue when we exercise will be answered.

If the answer is yes it can lead to the production of therapeutics that contain this hormone or contain things that tweak the cells in the muscles to produce this healthy protein. The restriction of calories in addition to certain plant nutrients (green tea, berberine, resveratrol) can cause PGC1 alpha synthesis. This can increase and support the production of Irisin during exercise.

Cleaner Cells and More Exercise

Leaner cells are the potential benefit of exercise. Another is cleaner cells. There is a report that goes into the activation of authopagy, a process of house cleaning the cells in muscles that are exercised. This was published in Health Journal Volume 9, Number 5, "Younger-acting Cells: A Balance to Clear the Way."

A Texas Southwestern Medical Center research team did some brief research on the cellular makeup of mice. They discovered that the process of getting rid of old components (proteins, mitochondria etc.)

and replacing them with new ones was much more prevalent in mice that were exercising regularly.

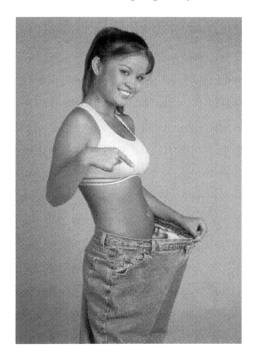

The method is a bit complex, but the link was made between improvements in metabolism and authopagy that was exercise induced. As an example cleaning out the old cells helps to alter the old cells with poor metabolism of glucose to younger cells that have a metabolic balance that is healthy. Organs like the liver and pancreas also had improvements in metabolism after exercise.

The main element of the hormone diet is exercise and foods that are low in carbs.

Exercise and a Diet Low in Carbs – A Preliminary Shopping List

Produce

Consume a variety of low sugar fruits and non starchy vegetables like:

Cabbage, spinach, lettuce (salad greens)

Bok Choy, kale, collard greens, Swiss or other chard (other leafy greens)

Cilantro, parsley, basil (herbs)

Tomatoes, cucumbers, sprouts, radishes (other salad vegetables)

Cauliflower, okra, Brussels sprouts, green beans, broccoli, asparagus, avocado (other green vegetables)

Mushrooms, artichokes, eggplant, green onions, peppers, summer squashes (other non starchy vegetables)

If you can eat fruit, small peaches, melons and berries are ideal choices.

Eggs, Seafood, Poultry and Meat

Any of these are okay. Liver and oysters do not have a lot of carbs and eggs are very nutritious. There are some diets that recommend eating moderate amounts in the initial stages.

Dairy

Sugar free yogurt, ricotta, cheeses, sour cream, full fat cottage cheese, butter and cream

Oils and Fats

A lot of authors of low carb diets state that foods with coconut oil and butter (high saturated fats) do not pose a problem in diets that are low carb while others stay away from it altogether. A lot state that these oils that have omega 6 fats like sunflower, most safflower, corn and soy should be avoided. So should partially hydrogenated oils.

Olive oil

Coconut oil

Sunflower and high mono safflower oils

Nut oils and sesame oils can be used in small amounts as flavoring

High fat foods like cream, avocados, seeds, nut butters and nuts

Frozen Foods

Frozen berries, vegetables, fish and meats are ideal to have on hand

Canned Goods

Coconut milk, olives, black coy beans and canned vegetables

Seeds and Nuts

A lot of the seeds and nuts (along with butters made from them) can be consumed, just watch the carbs. Coconut meal, flour, almond and flax are great for baking just ensure the ingredients are fresh. A lot of diets don't include legumes which includes peanuts.

Condiments

Sugar free preserves and jams, sugar free pickle relish, hot sauce, spices, bouillon or broth, pesto sauce, soy sauce, sugar free salad dressings (no soy oil), full fat mayo (no soy oil) and mustard

Other:

Pork rinds

Hemp milk, rice, almond and unsweetened soy

Unsweetened coconut

Low carb tortillas

Unsweetened cocoa and chocolate powder

With a diet that is moderate you can include limited amounts of fruit, barley, quinoa, rice, high fiber breads, beans and al dents pasta.

Aisles to Stay Out Of

The aisles that you should not even venture down are processed foods, baking supplies, pasta, candy, bread, crackers, cookies and baked goods.

ABOUT THE AUTHOR

The search for the perfect solution to health is always at the forefront of many people's minds and this includes Anna Gracey. She has tried many diets and done a lot of research which has led her to her latest find, the hormone diet. It is clear that she went all out with the research as a lot of the studies that she has read have been cited in support of the diet.

She implores the reader to look at all aspects of what is being said and then make the ultimate decision on what to do in the long run. She even close with information on the latest study being done on a particular hormone known as Irisin and how with regular exercises it can make our cells even better and literally help clean out the weak ones.

The requirements for the diet are not that extreme so persons will not be stressed by the fact that they have to give up everything that they grew up eating. If your family was really health conscious most of the restricted items would never have been eaten anyway. Anna stands behind this diet and feels that it is the solution to most of our problems.